South Beach Diet Easy Guide for Beginners

Making the Most of the South Beach Diet

By

Kenneth Achille

Table of Contents

CHAPTER 1

Introduction to the South Beach Diet

1.1 What is the South Beach Diet

The South Beach Diet is a popular and effective weight loss program developed by Dr. Arthur Agatston, a cardiologist, in the early 2000s. It is not just a short-term diet but also a lifestyle approach to healthy eating. The primary focus of the South Beach Diet is to help individuals make better food choices by incorporating the right balance of carbohydrates, lean proteins, and healthy fats into their meals.

Unlike some restrictive diets, the South Beach Diet does not eliminate entire food groups but instead emphasizes choosing the right types of carbohydrates and fats. It aims to stabilize blood sugar levels, reduce cravings, and promote sustainable weight loss.

The South Beach Diet is divided into three phases, each with a specific purpose and recommended food choices. Phase 1 is the most restrictive, focusing on rapid weight loss by eliminating high-glycemic index carbohydrates and sugars. Phase 2 allows for the gradual reintroduction of certain carbohydrates while continuing to promote weight loss. Phase 3 is the maintenance phase, emphasizing a balanced diet and long-term healthy eating habits.

In addition to weight loss, the South Beach Diet is known to improve overall health markers, including cholesterol levels, blood pressure, and insulin resistance. It has gained popularity due to its practical approach, flexibility, and emphasis on whole, nutrient-dense foods.

Throughout this guide, we will provide you with the necessary information and tools to start your journey with the South Beach Diet, making it an easy and accessible resource for beginners seeking a healthier lifestyle and weight management.

1.2 How Does the South Beach Diet Work

The South Beach Diet works by focusing on the quality of carbohydrates and fats consumed, rather than simply counting calories. It aims to regulate blood sugar levels and insulin response, which helps control hunger, reduce cravings, and promote weight loss. Here's how the diet works:

Phase 1: Kickstart Your Weight Loss

- During this phase, which typically lasts for two weeks, you eliminate most carbohydrates and sugars from your diet.

- The goal is to stabilize blood sugar levels and reduce cravings for unhealthy foods.

- You can consume lean proteins, vegetables, legumes, and healthy fats.

Phase 2: Steady Weight Loss

- In this phase, you gradually reintroduce certain carbohydrates, such as whole grains and fruits, while continuing to lose weight.

- The emphasis is on choosing low-glycemic index carbs, which have a minimal impact on blood sugar levels.

- You continue to include lean proteins, vegetables, legumes, and healthy fats in your meals.

Phase 3: Maintenance and Lifelong Healthy Eating

CHAPTER 2

Getting Started with the South Beach Diet

2.1 Setting Goals and Expectations

Before starting the South Beach Diet, it's important to set realistic goals and establish clear expectations for yourself. Here are some steps to help you get started:

1. Assess Your Current Situation: Take stock of your current weight, health, and lifestyle. Determine how much weight you want to lose and what specific health goals you have, such as improving cholesterol

levels or increasing energy
levels.

2. Set Realistic Goals: Set
   achievable and realistic goals
   for yourself. It's generally
   recommended to aim for a
   gradual and steady weight loss
   of 1-2 pounds per week. Keep
   in mind that the South Beach
   Diet is not just about weight
   loss but also about improving
   overall health and establishing
   long-term healthy habits.

3. Make Your Goals Specific and
   Measurable: Instead of saying,
   "I want to lose weight," be
   specific about how much
   weight you want to lose and by
   when. For example, "I want to
   lose 10 pounds in the next 8
   weeks."

4. Consider Non-Scale Goals: In addition to weight loss, think about other goals you want to achieve. These could include increased energy, improved fitness, better sleep, or better control of blood sugar levels.

5. Write Down Your Goals: Putting your goals in writing makes them more tangible and helps you stay focused. Keep a journal or create a vision board to remind yourself of your goals and track your progress.

6. Stay Positive and Realistic: Understand that weight loss is a journey with ups and downs. Be kind to yourself and celebrate small victories along the way. Remember that the South Beach Diet is a lifestyle

change and a long-term commitment to your health.

2.2 Understanding the Phases of the South Beach Diet

The South Beach Diet is divided into three phases, each with its own guidelines and objectives. Here's an overview of each phase:

Phase 1: Kickstart Your Weight Loss

- Duration: Typically lasts for two weeks.

- Objective: Stabilize blood sugar levels, reduce cravings, and jump-start weight loss.

- Food Choices: Lean proteins (e.g., chicken, fish, tofu), non-

CHAPTER 3

Phase 1: Kickstart Your Weight Loss

3.1 Overview of Phase 1

Phase 1 of the South Beach Diet is designed to kickstart your weight loss journey by stabilizing blood sugar levels, reducing cravings, and promoting rapid initial weight loss. This phase typically lasts for two weeks and is the most restrictive phase of the diet. Its primary focus is on eliminating high-glycemic index carbohydrates and sugars from your meals.

During Phase 1, you'll consume a variety of lean proteins, non-starchy vegetables, legumes, healthy fats, and sugar-free foods. By cutting out high-glycemic carbs and sugars, your body shifts to burning stored fat for energy, leading to weight loss.

3.2 Foods to Enjoy in Phase 1

In Phase 1, you have a wide range of food options that are nutritious and satisfying. Here are some foods you can enjoy:

1. Lean Proteins:

   - Skinless chicken breast

   - Turkey breast

   - Fish (such as salmon, cod, tuna)

   - Lean beef (such as sirloin, tenderloin)

- Tofu

- Eggs (including egg whites)

2. Non-Starchy Vegetables:

- Broccoli

- Spinach

- Cauliflower

- Asparagus

- Brussels sprouts

- Peppers

- Zucchini

- Cabbage

- Lettuce

- Cucumbers

3. Legumes:

- Lentils

- Black beans

- Chickpeas

- Edamame

4. Healthy Fats:

- Olive oil

- Avocados

- Nuts (such as almonds, walnuts, pistachios)

- Seeds (such as chia seeds, flaxseeds)

5. Low-Fat Dairy:

- Greek yogurt (unsweetened)

- Cottage cheese (low-fat)

- Reduced-fat cheese

6. Sugar-Free Foods:

- Sugar-free gelatin

- Sugar-free gum

- Sugar-free beverages
  (such as unsweetened tea
  or coffee)

It's important to note that portion sizes
and moderation are key in Phase 1.
Also, remember to drink plenty of
water to stay hydrated.

During Phase 1, it's recommended to
avoid high-glycemic index
carbohydrates, sugars, fruit, alcohol,
and certain types of fats. These
include items like white bread, rice,
pasta, potatoes, sugary snacks,
desserts, sweetened beverages, and
high-fat processed foods.

By enjoying a variety of lean proteins,
non-starchy vegetables, legumes, and

healthy fats, you'll provide your body with essential nutrients while kickstarting your weight loss journey in Phase 1 of the South Beach Diet.

3.3 Foods to Avoid in Phase 1

During Phase 1 of the South Beach Diet, it's important to avoid certain foods that can spike blood sugar levels and hinder weight loss progress. Here are the foods to avoid in Phase 1:

1. High-Glycemic Index Carbohydrates:

    - White bread

    - White rice

    - Pasta

- Potatoes

- Corn

- Cereal

- Processed grains

2. Sugars and Sweeteners:

- Regular sugar

- Honey

- Maple syrup

- Agave nectar

- Artificial sweeteners

3. Fruits:

- All fruits (including
  fresh, dried, and canned)
  are restricted in Phase 1.

4. Alcohol:

- All alcoholic beverages should be avoided during Phase 1.

5. Certain Types of Fats:

  - Trans fats (found in many processed and fried foods)

  - Saturated fats (found in fatty meats, full-fat dairy, and high-fat processed foods)

It's important to read food labels carefully to identify hidden sugars and avoid products that contain them. Focus on whole, unprocessed foods and choose items that are low in added sugars.

Remember, Phase 1 is a temporary phase, and these restrictions are in place to help stabilize blood sugar levels and promote rapid initial weight loss. In later phases, certain foods will be gradually reintroduced.

3.4 Sample Phase 1 Meal Plan

Here's a sample Phase 1 meal plan to give you an idea of how to structure your meals during this phase:

Day 1:

- Breakfast: Veggie omelet made with egg whites, spinach, bell peppers, and onions.

- Snack: Celery sticks with sugar-free peanut butter.

- Lunch: Grilled chicken breast with steamed broccoli and a side of mixed greens.

- Snack: Hard-boiled eggs.

- Dinner: Baked salmon with roasted asparagus and a side salad with olive oil dressing.

- Snack: Sugar-free gelatin.

Day 2:

- Breakfast: Greek yogurt with a handful of nuts and seeds.

- Snack: Sliced cucumbers with hummus.

- Lunch: Turkey lettuce wraps filled with lean turkey breast, lettuce, and sliced tomatoes.

- Snack: Sugar-free protein shake.

- Dinner: Grilled shrimp with sautéed zucchini noodles and a side of steamed green beans.

- Snack: Sugar-free gum.

Remember to adjust portion sizes based on your individual needs and consult with a healthcare professional before starting any new diet or weight loss program.

3.5 Tips and Tricks for Phase 1 Success

Here are some helpful tips and tricks to ensure success during Phase 1 of the South Beach Diet:

1. Plan Your Meals: Take the time to plan your meals and snacks in advance. This will help you stay on track and avoid impulsive, unhealthy food choices.

2. Prep Ahead: Prepare your meals and snacks in advance, especially during busy days. Batch cook proteins, chop vegetables, and portion out snacks to have them readily available.

3. Stay Hydrated: Drink plenty of water throughout the day. Staying hydrated helps control hunger, supports digestion, and promotes overall health.

4. Read Labels: Be mindful of food labels and ingredients. Avoid foods that contain added sugars, high-fructose corn syrup, or unhealthy fats. Look for whole, unprocessed options.

5. Use Herbs and Spices: Enhance the flavors of your meals with herbs, spices, and seasonings.

They add taste without adding extra calories or sugars.

6. Practice Portion Control: Be mindful of portion sizes, especially for higher-calorie foods like nuts and seeds. Use measuring cups or a food scale to ensure accurate portions.

7. Focus on Lean Proteins: Prioritize lean proteins such as skinless chicken, turkey, fish, tofu, and eggs. They provide essential nutrients and help keep you feeling satisfied.

8. Embrace Non-Starchy Vegetables: Fill your plate with non-starchy vegetables like broccoli, spinach, peppers, and cauliflower. They are low in calories, high in fiber, and packed with nutrients.

9. Find Sugar-Free Alternatives: Look for sugar-free versions of products like gelatin, gum, and beverages to satisfy cravings without compromising Phase 1 guidelines.

10. Seek Support: Consider joining online communities, forums, or finding an accountability partner who is also following the South Beach Diet. Sharing experiences and getting support can be motivating and helpful.

11. Keep a Journal: Keep track of your meals, snacks, and how you feel throughout the day. This can help identify patterns, track progress, and provide insights into your eating habits.

12. Stay Active: Incorporate regular physical activity into

your routine. Exercise not only supports weight loss but also boosts mood, energy levels, and overall well-being.

Phase 1 is temporary, and as you progress through the diet, more food options will be introduced. Stay committed, be patient, and celebrate your successes along the way.

CHAPTER 4

Phase 2: Steady Weight Loss

4.1 Overview of Phase 2

Phase 2 of the South Beach Diet is designed to promote steady weight loss while gradually reintroducing certain carbohydrates and fruits into your eating plan. This phase typically begins after completing Phase 1 and continues until you reach your desired weight loss goal.

The main objective of Phase 2 is to find the right balance of carbohydrates that don't cause significant spikes in blood sugar levels. By adding these "good carbs" and fruits back into your diet, you'll continue to lose weight at a steady pace while expanding your food options.

4.2 Adding Good Carbs and Fruits

During Phase 2, you'll introduce good carbohydrates and fruits back into your meals. These carbs have a lower glycemic index, meaning they have a lesser impact on blood sugar levels. Here are some examples of good carbs and fruits to include in Phase 2:

Good Carbohydrates:

- Whole grains: Quinoa, brown rice, whole wheat bread, whole grain pasta, oatmeal.

- Legumes: Black beans, chickpeas, lentils, kidney beans.

- Starchy vegetables: Sweet potatoes, butternut squash, peas, corn.

Fruits:

- Berries: Strawberries, blueberries, raspberries.

- Apples

- Oranges

- Melons: Watermelon, cantaloupe, honeydew.

- Kiwi

- Grapefruit

It's important to note that portion control remains crucial during Phase 2. Be mindful of the quantity of carbohydrates and fruits you consume, and adjust according to your individual needs and weight loss goals. It's always a good idea to listen to your body and observe how different foods affect your energy levels, hunger, and overall well-being.

The South Beach Diet is a lifestyle approach to eating, and Phase 2 is about finding a sustainable balance that works for you. Regularly monitor your progress, make adjustments as needed, and continue incorporating lean proteins, non-starchy vegetables, healthy fats, and good carbohydrates into your meals for optimal results.

4.3 Sample Phase 2 Meal Plan

Here's a sample Phase 2 meal plan to give you an idea of how to structure your meals during this phase:

Day 1:

- Breakfast: Scrambled eggs with vegetables (such as spinach, mushrooms, and peppers) and a slice of whole wheat toast.

- Snack: Greek yogurt with mixed berries.

- Lunch: Grilled chicken salad with mixed greens, cherry tomatoes, cucumbers, and a sprinkle of feta cheese.

- Snack: Carrot sticks with hummus.

- Dinner: Baked salmon with quinoa and steamed asparagus.

- Snack: Apple slices with almond butter.

Day 2:

- Breakfast: Oatmeal cooked with almond milk, topped with sliced bananas and a sprinkle of cinnamon.

- Snack: Hard-boiled eggs.

- Lunch: Turkey wrap with whole wheat tortilla, turkey breast, lettuce, tomatoes, and avocado slices. Serve with a side of carrot and celery sticks.

- Snack: Mixed nuts (portion-controlled).

- Dinner: Grilled shrimp skewers with roasted sweet potatoes and a side of sautéed broccoli.

- Snack: Greek yogurt with a drizzle of honey.

Adjust portion sizes based on your individual needs and consult with a healthcare professional before starting any new diet or weight loss program. Feel free to modify the meal plan to suit your preferences and dietary requirements.

During Phase 2, continue incorporating lean proteins, non-starchy vegetables, healthy fats, and good carbohydrates into your meals. Focus on whole, unprocessed foods, and make sure to stay hydrated by drinking plenty of water throughout the day.

4.4 Tips for Maintaining Weight Loss in Phase 2

Maintaining weight loss in Phase 2 of the South Beach Diet is an important step towards your long-term goals. Here are some tips to help you stay on track and continue your success during this phase:

1. Monitor Portion Sizes: Even though you're reintroducing good carbs and fruits, it's essential to maintain portion control. Be mindful of the quantity of food you consume and avoid overeating.

2. Focus on Balanced Meals: Create well-rounded meals that include lean proteins, non-starchy vegetables, good carbs, and a source of healthy fats. This combination will help you

feel satisfied, maintain stable
blood sugar levels, and support
weight loss.

3. Listen to Your Body: Pay
attention to your body's hunger
and fullness cues. Eat until
you're satisfied, not overly
stuffed. Practice mindful eating
and be present during meals to
avoid mindless snacking.

4. Prioritize Fiber: Continue
incorporating fiber-rich foods
into your meals, such as non-
starchy vegetables, whole
grains, and legumes. Fiber
helps promote satiety, aids in
digestion, and supports overall
health.

5. Hydrate Well: Stay hydrated by
drinking an adequate amount of
water throughout the day.

Water helps control appetite, supports digestion, and promotes overall well-being. Aim to drink at least 8 cups (64 ounces) of water daily.

6. Engage in Regular Physical Activity: Maintain an active lifestyle by incorporating regular exercise into your routine. Physical activity not only aids in weight management but also boosts mood, improves fitness, and supports overall health.

7. Plan and Prepare Meals: Continue planning your meals and snacks in advance to stay organized and make healthier choices. Prepare meals at home whenever possible to have better control over the ingredients and portion sizes.

8. Monitor Progress and Adjust as
    Needed: Regularly monitor
    your progress, including
    weight, measurements, and
    overall well-being. If you hit a
    weight loss plateau or feel
    stuck, consider reassessing your
    food choices, portion sizes, or
    increasing physical activity
    levels.

9. Practice Mindful Eating: Slow
    down while eating and savor
    each bite. Be aware of your
    body's hunger and fullness
    signals. Avoid distractions like
    screens or eating on the go, as it
    can lead to overeating or
    mindless snacking.

10. Seek Support and
    Accountability: Stay connected
    with support systems, such as
    online communities or

accountability partners. Sharing experiences, tips, and challenges can help you stay motivated and focused on your weight loss journey.

Phase 2 is a crucial part of the South Beach Diet where you continue to make progress towards your weight loss goals. Be patient, stay consistent, and embrace the healthy habits you've developed. Celebrate your achievements and continue making mindful choices for long-term success.

CHAPTER 5

Phase 3: Maintenance and Lifelong Healthy Eating

5.1 Overview of Phase 3

Phase 3 of the South Beach Diet focuses on maintaining your weight loss and adopting a balanced eating pattern for life. It is the final phase of the diet and is designed to help you sustain the healthy habits you've developed during Phases 1 and 2.

In Phase 3, you'll continue to follow the principles of the South Beach Diet but with more flexibility and a wider variety of food choices. The emphasis is on making long-term, sustainable changes to your eating habits and lifestyle.

5.2 Transitioning to a Balanced Diet

During Phase 3, you'll transition to a balanced diet that includes a variety of nutrient-dense foods. Here are some key principles to keep in mind:

1. Maintain Portion Control: Continue practicing portion control to ensure you're consuming appropriate amounts of food. Be mindful of your hunger and fullness cues and avoid overeating.

2. Choose Whole, Unprocessed Foods: opt for whole grains,

lean proteins, non-starchy
vegetables, fruits, healthy fats,
and low-fat dairy products.
These foods provide essential
nutrients while promoting
overall health.

3. Focus on Quality
    Carbohydrates: Include
    carbohydrates with a low
    glycemic index, such as whole
    grains, legumes, and starchy
    vegetables. These carbs are
    digested more slowly, helping
    to stabilize blood sugar levels
    and provide sustained energy.

4. Prioritize Lean Proteins:
    Include lean proteins like
    skinless poultry, fish, lean cuts
    of beef, tofu, and legumes.
    These protein sources are lower
    in saturated fats and can help
    you feel full and satisfied.

5. Emphasize Non-Starchy Vegetables: Continue to incorporate non-starchy vegetables like leafy greens, peppers, broccoli, and cauliflower into your meals. These vegetables are rich in fiber, vitamins, and minerals while being low in calories.

6. Include Healthy Fats: Choose sources of healthy fats such as olive oil, avocados, nuts, and seeds. These fats provide essential fatty acids and help you feel satisfied.

7. Practice Mindful Eating: Continue practicing mindful eating by being present during meals, eating slowly, and paying attention to your body's hunger and fullness cues. Enjoy your food and savor the flavors.

8. Regular Physical Activity:
    Maintain an active lifestyle by
    engaging in regular physical
    activity. Aim for a combination
    of cardiovascular exercises,
    strength training, and flexibility
    exercises for overall fitness and
    well-being.

9. Occasional Indulgences: Allow
    yourself the occasional
    indulgence in moderation.
    Enjoy your favorite treats or
    special meals on occasion, but
    remember to maintain balance
    and portion control.

10. Long-Term Sustainability:
    Remember that Phase 3 is
    about adopting a sustainable
    eating pattern for life. Use the
    principles you've learned
    during the South Beach Diet to

make healthy choices and maintain your weight loss.

Phase 3 is a continuation of the healthy habits you've developed in the earlier phases. It's an opportunity to maintain your weight loss, enjoy a wide variety of nutritious foods, and make lifelong changes for better health and well-being.

5.3 Sample Phase 3 Meal Plan

Here's a sample Phase 3 meal plan to give you an idea of how to structure your meals during this phase:

Day 1:

- Breakfast: Vegetable omelet made with whole eggs, spinach, mushrooms, and tomatoes.

Serve with a side of whole grain toast.

- Snack: Greek yogurt with mixed berries and a sprinkle of granola.

- Lunch: Grilled chicken salad with mixed greens, cherry tomatoes, cucumbers, avocado slices, and a drizzle of olive oil dressing.

- Snack: Carrot sticks with hummus.

- Dinner: Baked salmon with quinoa pilaf and roasted Brussels sprouts.

- Snack: Apple slices with almond butter.

Day 2:

- Breakfast: Overnight oats made with rolled oats, almond milk, chia seeds, and topped with sliced bananas and a sprinkle of cinnamon.

- Snack: Hard-boiled eggs.

- Lunch: Turkey and vegetable wrap with whole wheat tortilla, turkey breast, lettuce, tomatoes, cucumbers, and a spread of hummus. Serve with a side of mixed fruit.

- Snack: Mixed nuts (portion-controlled).

- Dinner: Grilled shrimp skewers with brown rice, roasted sweet potatoes, and a side of steamed broccoli.

- Snack: Greek yogurt with a drizzle of honey and sliced almonds.

Adjust portion sizes based on your individual needs and consult with a healthcare professional before starting any new diet or weight maintenance plan. Feel free to modify the meal plan to suit your preferences and dietary requirements.

During Phase 3, continue focusing on balanced meals that include lean proteins, whole grains, non-starchy vegetables, fruits, and healthy fats. Enjoy a wide variety of foods and savor the flavors while practicing portion control and mindful eating.

5.4 Strategies for Long-Term Success

Maintaining long-term success with the South Beach Diet and adopting a healthy lifestyle requires strategies and ongoing commitment. Here are some strategies to help you sustain your progress beyond Phase 3:

1. Stay Consistent: Stick to the principles of the South Beach Diet and continue making healthy food choices consistently. Consistency is key to maintaining weight loss and achieving long-term success.

2. Practice Portion Control: Be mindful of portion sizes to prevent overeating. Use measuring cups, a food scale, or visual cues to help you estimate appropriate portion sizes.

3. Focus on Whole Foods: Emphasize whole, unprocessed foods in your meals. Choose lean proteins, whole grains, non-starchy vegetables, fruits, and healthy fats. These foods provide essential nutrients and support overall health.

4. Practice Mindful Eating: Slow down and be present during meals. Pay attention to your body's hunger and fullness signals. Eat slowly, chew your food thoroughly, and savor the flavors. This can help prevent overeating and promote better digestion.

5. Prioritize Regular Exercise: Engage in regular physical activity to maintain weight loss, improve fitness, and support overall well-being. Find

activities you enjoy and make them a part of your routine.

6. Manage Stress: Stress can impact your eating habits and overall well-being. Find healthy ways to manage stress, such as practicing relaxation techniques, engaging in hobbies, or seeking social support.

7. Build a Support System: Surround yourself with supportive individuals who understand and encourage your healthy lifestyle goals. Joining online communities, finding an accountability partner, or participating in support groups can provide motivation and support.

8. Monitor Progress: Continue monitoring your progress beyond Phase 3. Keep track of your weight, measurements, and overall well-being. Regular self-assessment can help you stay aware of any changes and make necessary adjustments.

9. Make Healthy Habits Sustainable: Incorporate healthy habits into your daily life. Choose activities and eating patterns that you enjoy and can maintain in the long run. This is not a temporary diet but a lifelong commitment to health.

10. Celebrate Non-Scale Victories: Focus on more than just the number on the scale. Celebrate non-scale victories, such as increased energy, improved

fitness, better sleep, or healthier habits. Recognize and reward yourself for all the positive changes you've made.

Maintaining long-term success is about finding a balance that works for you and making sustainable lifestyle changes. Be patient, stay committed, and embrace the healthy habits you've developed. With the right strategies and mindset, you can achieve lasting success with the South Beach Diet.

CHAPTER 6

Making the Most of the South Beach Diet

6.1 Incorporating Exercise into Your Routine

Exercise is an essential component of a healthy lifestyle and can greatly enhance the benefits of the South Beach Diet. Here are some tips for incorporating exercise into your routine:

1. Choose Activities You Enjoy: Find physical activities that you genuinely enjoy. Whether it's jogging, dancing, cycling, swimming, or playing a sport, engaging in activities you love

will make exercise more enjoyable and sustainable.

2. Start Slowly and Gradually Increase Intensity: If you're new to exercise or haven't been active for a while, start with low-impact activities and gradually increase the intensity and duration over time. This approach helps prevent injuries and allows your body to adjust.

3. Set Realistic Goals: Set achievable goals for your exercise routine. Aim for at least 150 minutes of moderate-intensity aerobic activity or 75 minutes of vigorous-intensity aerobic activity per week, along with strength training exercises twice a week. Start with smaller goals and build up as your fitness improves.

4. Mix Up Your Routine: Keep your exercise routine interesting by incorporating a variety of activities. Alternate between cardiovascular exercises (such as jogging, cycling, or swimming) and strength training exercises (such as weightlifting or bodyweight exercises) to work different muscle groups and improve overall fitness.

5. Find Opportunities for Daily Movement: Look for opportunities to incorporate more movement into your daily life. Take the stairs instead of the elevator, park farther away from your destination to get in extra steps, or take short breaks throughout the day to stretch and move around.

6. Schedule Exercise Sessions:
Treat exercise as an important
appointment in your calendar.
Set aside dedicated time for
physical activity and stick to
your schedule. Consistency is
key to reaping the benefits of
exercise.

7. Mix Cardiovascular and
Strength Training: Combine
cardiovascular exercises with
strength training to maximize
the benefits. Cardiovascular
exercises help burn calories and
improve cardiovascular health,
while strength training helps
build lean muscle, increase
metabolism, and improve
overall body composition.

8. Listen to Your Body: Pay
attention to your body's signals
and adjust your exercise routine

accordingly. If you experience pain or discomfort, modify or choose alternative activities. Rest and recovery are equally important for your overall well-being.

9. Seek Professional Guidance if Needed: If you're new to exercise or have specific health concerns, consider consulting with a fitness professional or healthcare provider. They can provide personalized guidance, create a tailored exercise plan, and ensure you're exercising safely.

10. Stay Motivated: Find ways to stay motivated and accountable. Set goals, track your progress, reward yourself for achieving milestones, and seek support

from friends, family, or fitness communities.

Regular exercise not only supports weight management but also improves cardiovascular health, boosts mood, increases energy levels, and enhances overall well-being. By incorporating exercise into your routine alongside the South Beach Diet, you can optimize your results and enjoy a healthier lifestyle.

6.2 Tips for Dining Out and Social Events

Navigating dining out and social events while following the South Beach Diet can be challenging, but with some preparation and mindful choices, you can stay on track. Here are some tips to help you make the most of these situations:

1. Plan Ahead: If you know you'll be dining out or attending a social event, plan your meals and snacks for the day accordingly. Eat a balanced meal before the event to avoid arriving hungry and making impulsive food choices.

2. Research the Menu: Before going to a restaurant, check the menu online if available. Look for healthier options that align with the South Beach Diet principles. Choose grilled or baked lean proteins, salads with dressing on the side, and non-starchy vegetable sides.

3. Customize Your Order: Don't be afraid to ask for

modifications to suit your dietary needs. Request dressings or sauces on the side, substitute high-carb sides with extra vegetables or a side salad, and ask for grilled or steamed preparations.

4. Watch Portion Sizes: Restaurant portions can be larger than necessary. Consider sharing a meal with a friend or ask for a to-go box to portion out half of your meal before you start eating. This helps avoid overeating and allows you to enjoy leftovers later.

5. Be Mindful of Hidden Ingredients: Be cautious of hidden ingredients that may not be listed on the menu. Ask about cooking oils, added sugars, or sauces that may be

used. Choose simpler preparations to avoid unwanted additives.

6. Enjoy Healthy Appetizers: Instead of reaching for fried or high-calorie appetizers, opt for healthier choices like a salad, vegetable-based soup, or grilled shrimp cocktail.

7. Stay Hydrated: Drink water or unsweetened beverages instead of sugary cocktails or sodas. If you choose to consume alcohol, opt for lower-sugar options like dry wine or spirits mixed with soda water and fresh lime.

8. Bring a Dish: If you're attending a potluck or social gathering, offer to bring a dish that aligns with the South Beach Diet. This way, you'll

have a healthier option available and can share it with others.

9. Practice Mindful Eating: Slow down and savor each bite. Pay attention to your body's hunger and fullness cues. Listen to your body and stop eating when you feel satisfied, even if there is food remaining on your plate.

10. Focus on Socializing: Shift the focus of social events from just the food to enjoying the company of others. Engage in conversations, participate in activities, and enjoy the overall experience beyond the food.

11. Don't Be Too Hard on Yourself: Remember that occasional indulgences are part of a balanced lifestyle. If you

choose to enjoy a treat or
deviate from the South Beach
Diet guidelines at a special
event, do so in moderation and
get back on track with your
healthy eating habits afterward.

By being prepared, making mindful
choices, and finding a balance
between enjoying social events and
following the South Beach Diet
principles, you can successfully
navigate dining out and social
gatherings while still progressing
towards your health goals.

6.3 Overcoming Challenges and Staying Motivated

Overcoming challenges and staying
motivated are crucial for long-term

success with the South Beach Diet. Here are some tips to help you overcome obstacles and maintain your motivation:

1. Set Realistic and Specific Goals: Set clear and achievable goals that are specific to you. Whether it's weight loss, improved health markers, or increased energy levels, having specific goals helps you stay focused and motivated.

2. Track Your Progress: Keep track of your progress to see how far you've come. Monitor your weight, measurements, or take photos to visually see the changes in your body. Celebrate your achievements along the way to stay motivated.

3. Find Support: Surround
    yourself with a supportive
    network of family, friends, or
    online communities who share
    similar health goals. Lean on
    them for support,
    accountability, and
    encouragement during
    challenging times.

4. Focus on Non-Scale Victories:
    Don't solely rely on the number
    on the scale as a measure of
    success. Acknowledge and
    celebrate non-scale victories
    like increased energy, improved
    sleep, or positive changes in
    your overall well-being.

5. Stay Educated: Continue
    learning about nutrition,
    healthy eating, and the science
    behind the South Beach Diet.
    Understanding the principles

and benefits of the diet can reinforce your motivation and commitment to a healthier lifestyle.

6. Find Healthy Food Swaps: Explore creative ways to make healthier versions of your favorite dishes. Look for South Beach Diet-friendly recipes or experiment with ingredient substitutions to enjoy your favorite meals while staying on track.

7. Prepare for Challenges: Anticipate and plan for potential challenges or obstacles that may arise. Whether it's a busy schedule, social events, or cravings, having a plan in place can help you navigate these situations more effectively.

8. Practice Mindfulness: Cultivate mindfulness in your eating habits. Pay attention to your body's hunger and fullness cues, eat slowly, and savor the flavors of your food. Mindful eating helps you make conscious choices and prevents overeating.

9. Reward Yourself: Celebrate your achievements with non-food rewards. Treat yourself to a massage, a new workout outfit, or a relaxing day off. Rewarding yourself reinforces positive behaviors and keeps you motivated.

10. Stay Positive and Practice Self-Compassion: Be kind to yourself throughout your journey. Don't dwell on slip-ups or setbacks. Instead, focus

on the progress you've made
and recommit to your goals
with a positive mindset.

11. Stay Active and Try New
Activities: Keep your exercise
routine interesting by trying
new activities or workouts.
Explore different types of
exercises, classes, or outdoor
activities to keep your body and
mind engaged.

12. Visualize Success: Imagine
yourself achieving your goals
and living a healthier lifestyle.
Visualizing success can help
you stay motivated and focused
on your long-term vision.

CHAPTER 7

How to Customize the South Beach Diet to your Preferences

Customizing the South Beach Diet to your preferences can help make it a sustainable and enjoyable eating plan. Here are some tips on how to personalize the diet:

1. Review the Food List: Familiarize yourself with the approved food list for each phase of the South Beach Diet. Identify foods that you enjoy and feel comfortable incorporating into your meals.

2. Modify Recipes: Adapt South Beach Diet recipes to suit your

taste preferences and dietary needs. Experiment with different seasonings, herbs, and spices to add flavor to your meals. Substitute ingredients when necessary to accommodate food allergies or sensitivities.

3. Adjust Portion Sizes: Tailor portion sizes based on your individual needs and goals. Consider your activity level, energy requirements, and hunger cues to determine appropriate serving sizes. Remember that portion control plays a significant role in weight management.

4. Personalize the Phases: If you feel that a particular phase of the South Beach Diet is too restrictive or not aligned with

your goals, you can modify it slightly. For example, you may choose to spend more time in Phase 1 or progress through the phases at a slower pace. Just ensure you're still following the core principles of the diet.

5. Include Favorite Foods: Incorporate your favorite foods into the South Beach Diet within the framework of the diet's guidelines. For example, if you enjoy a particular fruit or whole grain that isn't included in a specific phase, you can introduce it in moderation and monitor how it affects your progress.

6. Seek Professional Guidance: If you have specific dietary restrictions, medical conditions, or concerns, consult with a

registered dietitian or healthcare professional. They can provide personalized recommendations and guidance to help you customize the South Beach Diet according to your individual needs.

7. Focus on Sustainable Habits: Use the South Beach Diet as a foundation for developing sustainable eating habits. Incorporate whole, unprocessed foods, prioritize lean proteins, non-starchy vegetables, and healthy fats. Make the South Beach Diet principles a part of your long-term healthy lifestyle.

8. Enjoy Flexibility: While the South Beach Diet provides guidelines and structure, remember that flexibility is

key. Life happens, and there may be occasions where you deviate from the diet. Don't be too hard on yourself and aim for consistency rather than perfection.

9. Experiment and Explore: Continually explore new recipes, flavors, and ingredients that fit within the South Beach Diet framework. This can help you discover new foods you enjoy and keep your meals interesting and diverse.

10. Listen to Your Body: Pay attention to how different foods make you feel. Observe how they affect your energy levels, digestion, and overall well-being. Adjust your food choices accordingly to create a personalized eating plan that

supports your health and preferences.

The South Beach Diet is a flexible approach to eating, and personalizing it can make it more enjoyable and sustainable for you. By understanding the core principles and adapting them to fit your preferences and needs, you can create a customized version of the diet that works best for you.

CHAPTER 8

Handling plateaus and weight loss stalls

Hitting a weight loss plateau can be frustrating, but it's a common occurrence in any weight loss journey. Here are some strategies to overcome a plateau and continue making progress:

1. Assess Your Habits: Take a closer look at your eating and exercise habits. Are there any areas where you may have become less consistent or have slipped back into old patterns? Be honest with yourself and

identify any areas that may need improvement.

2. Reevaluate Portion Sizes: Portion control plays a crucial role in weight management. Assess your portion sizes to ensure you're still consuming appropriate amounts of food. It's possible that portion sizes may have increased over time without you realizing it.

3. Adjust Caloric Intake: As you lose weight, your body's caloric needs may change. Reassess your caloric intake to ensure it aligns with your current weight and activity level. You may need to slightly reduce your calorie intake to break through the plateau.

4. Increase Physical Activity: If you've been consistent with your exercise routine, consider adding more intensity or duration to your workouts. Incorporate strength training exercises to build lean muscle, which can help boost metabolism and break through plateaus.

5. Try New Exercises: Shake up your exercise routine by trying new activities or workouts. Your body may have become accustomed to your current routine, causing a plateau. Introducing new exercises can challenge your muscles and jumpstart your progress.

6. Review Your Food Choices: Take a closer look at the foods you're consuming. Are there

any hidden sources of added sugars or high-calorie ingredients that may be hindering your progress? Be mindful of your food choices and make adjustments if necessary.

7. Consider Meal Timing: Experiment with the timing of your meals and snacks. Some individuals find that adjusting meal frequency or incorporating intermittent fasting can help break through plateaus. Consult with a healthcare professional before making any drastic changes to your eating pattern.

8. Manage Stress: Chronic stress can impact weight loss progress. Implement stress management techniques such as

meditation, deep breathing
exercises, or engaging in
activities that help you relax.
Adequate sleep is also crucial
for managing stress and
supporting weight loss.

9. Stay Hydrated: Ensure you're
drinking enough water
throughout the day. Hydration
is important for overall health
and can aid in weight loss.
Sometimes, thirst can be
mistaken for hunger, leading to
increased calorie intake.

10. Stay Consistent and Patient:
Remember that weight loss
plateaus are normal and part of
the journey. Stay consistent
with your healthy habits,
remain patient, and trust the
process. Stay focused on the
overall improvements in your

well-being, not just the number on the scale.

If you've tried these strategies and are still struggling to break through a plateau, consider consulting with a registered dietitian or healthcare professional. They can provide personalized guidance and help identify any underlying factors that may be hindering your progress.

Keep in mind that sustainable weight loss is a gradual process. Celebrate your achievements along the way and focus on creating a healthy lifestyle that supports long-term well-being.

CHAPTER 9

Side Effects or Risks Associated with the South Beach Diet

While the South Beach Diet is generally considered safe for most individuals, it's important to be aware of potential side effects or risks. Here are some considerations to keep in mind:

1. Ketosis and Initial Side Effects: During Phase 1 of the South Beach Diet, some individuals may enter a state of ketosis, where the body primarily burns fat for fuel. This transition may cause temporary side effects

such as headache, fatigue, dizziness, and constipation. These symptoms usually subside as the body adapts to the diet.

2. Nutrient Deficiencies: If the diet is not well-balanced or followed incorrectly, there is a risk of nutrient deficiencies. This can occur if you're not consuming a variety of foods from different food groups. It's important to ensure you're getting adequate nutrients, including vitamins, minerals, and fiber, from a variety of food sources.

3. Restrictive Nature: The South Beach Diet can be restrictive, particularly during Phase 1. Some individuals may find it challenging to sustain such

restrictions long-term. It's important to find a balance that suits your preferences and lifestyle while still adhering to the core principles of the diet.

4. Individual Variations: Each person's response to the South Beach Diet may vary. Some individuals may experience more significant weight loss or changes in health markers, while others may not see the same level of results. It's important to focus on overall health improvements rather than comparing yourself to others.

5. Medical Considerations: If you have any underlying medical conditions, such as diabetes, kidney disease, or heart disease, or if you're taking medications,

it's essential to consult with a healthcare professional before starting the South Beach Diet. They can provide guidance on how to adapt the diet to your specific needs.

6. Individual Sensitivities: Some individuals may have sensitivities or allergies to specific foods that are included in the South Beach Diet. If you experience adverse reactions or discomfort after consuming certain foods, it's important to identify and avoid those triggers.

7. Psychological Considerations: Like any diet, the South Beach Diet may trigger emotional or psychological challenges for some individuals, especially if there is a history of disordered

eating or a negative relationship with food. It's important to approach the diet with a balanced mindset and prioritize overall well-being.

It's always recommended to consult with a healthcare professional, such as a registered dietitian or doctor, before starting any new diet or weight loss program. They can assess your individual needs, provide personalized guidance, and monitor your progress to ensure your safety and well-being.

CHAPTER 10

Staying Motivated and Overcoming Challenges

Staying motivated and committed to any diet can be challenging, and the South Beach Diet is no exception. However, with the right mindset and strategies, you can overcome obstacles and stay on track to achieve your goals. Here are some tips to help you stay motivated and overcome challenges on the South Beach Diet:

1. Set Realistic Goals: Start by setting realistic and achievable goals for yourself. Break down your larger goal into smaller

milestones and celebrate your progress along the way. This will help you stay motivated and give you a sense of accomplishment as you reach each milestone.

2. Find Your "Why": Take some time to reflect on why you started the South Beach Diet in the first place. Whether it's to improve your health, feel more confident, or have more energy, reminding yourself of your reasons can reignite your motivation during difficult times.

3. Create a Supportive Environment: Surround yourself with people who support your goals and understand your commitment to the South Beach Diet. Join

online communities, find an
accountability partner, or
involve your family and friends
in your journey. Having a
support system can make a
significant difference in staying
motivated and overcoming
challenges.

4. Plan Ahead: Planning ahead is
   crucial for success on the South
   Beach Diet. Set aside time each
   week to plan your meals, create
   a grocery list, and prepare
   meals in advance if possible.
   When you have healthy options
   readily available, you're less
   likely to give in to cravings or
   make impulsive food choices.

5. Find Enjoyable Recipes:
   Explore the wide variety of
   delicious recipes available that
   align with the South Beach Diet

principles. Look for creative ways to prepare your favorite foods while still staying within the guidelines. Discovering new recipes and flavors can keep your meals exciting and prevent boredom.

6. Track Your Progress: Keep a journal or use a tracking app to record your progress. This can include your food intake, exercise routine, and any positive changes you notice in your body or mindset. Tracking your progress helps you stay accountable and provides a visual representation of your achievements.

7. Stay Positive and Practice Self-Compassion: Remember that setbacks and challenges are a normal part of any journey. If

you slip up or deviate from the plan, don't beat yourself up. Instead, practice self-compassion and use it as an opportunity to learn and grow. Focus on the progress you've made and recommit to your goals.

8. Seek Inspiration and Motivation: Look for sources of inspiration to keep you motivated on your South Beach Diet journey. Read success stories, follow social media accounts that share healthy recipes and tips, or listen to podcasts or audiobooks related to health and wellness. Drawing inspiration from others can help you stay motivated and remind you that

you're not alone in your journey.

Staying motivated and overcoming challenges is a continuous process. Be patient with yourself, stay committed to your goals, and celebrate every small victory along the way. With perseverance and determination, you can achieve long-term success on the South Beach Diet.